DEFIANT DIE

From The Health

(Don Bee

To E, fondly /

Table of Contents

Contents

INTRODUCTION (1)

Here's my story.

My Doctor and the observing medical student stood with their mouths open, flummoxed.

It was my annual physical, and I had just told these two medical professionals that my diet includes lots of veggies, but also red meat, fat, butter and other dairy products…as well as beer and wine.

They were stumped. How could a 66 year old man with this kind of diet have such incredibly good numbers?

-My total cholesterol was 179. My good cholesterol was off the charts (105, when the range for a duck my age was 30-80). My bad cholesterol and triglycerides were at the very low end of their ranges. My PSA was minute (which is an extremely good thing).-

In fact, all of my numbers were the best ever.

I hadn't changed meds. I hadn't changed supplements. I hadn't exercised more. I still drank wine with dinner and had a couple of beers at night. I still ate fermented foods that were high in salt and other foods that were high in fat.

What had changed?

Here's what changed: I dropped carbs and sugars from my diet, and I ate as cleanly as was practical.

That's it, baby.

Is this paleo? Oh, maybe kinda-sorta. Paleo means eating what our ancestors ate, which excludes dairy, among other items, so I'm not strictly paleo. In fact, any paleo aspect to my diet is coincidental, but it is there. And straying from paleo isn't hurting me, as my physical condition testifies.

Dropping the carbs and sugar isn't complicated. It is easy to research which foods have these contents. Start reading labels, and you'll quickly uncover their hiding places. For example, take canned tomato juice, which you probably consider wholesome and healthy. Well it ain't so healthy because it has way too much sugar! Reading the label will inform you of this.

'Wait,' you say, 'does this mean no bread, pasta, pizza or ice cream?'

Yes, that is what it means.

'But, I couldn't give up those,' you protest. 'I love those foods!'

So do I, but it is a sacrifice I willingly make to feel good and to be healthy. Plus, I'm not lacking in really darned good foods. That's what this book is about.

If you want more convincing on why carbs (especially grains) and sugars are bad for you, read GRAIN BRAIN by Dr. David Perlmutter. The good Doctor will also educate you on why fat is good for you. Yes, that's right…good for you. Your brain *needs* fat. Fat also reduces your chance of developing Alzheimer's.

TIP: Go all in, or don't try this diet at all. No carbs, no sugars…period. The cravings will subside if you abstain. You must resist tasting 'just a little bit' when offered tempting foods, because while that little bit won't harm you, it will rejuvenate your yearnings. It took my well-meaning and generous wife (who doesn't follow this diet) some time to understand and accept this.

As far as eating cleanly, that means very little processed food, very little fast food and doing more of your own cooking.

'Whoa!' you protest? 'Cook more? ME?'

Calm down and consider this: people who do more cooking are healthier people because they are closer to their food. They know what the ingredients are, and those ingredients don't include unpronounceable chemicals. They get satisfaction from producing tasty meals, and they tend not to snack on crap.

For more information on the relationship between cooking your own food and improving your health, refer to COOKED, A Natural History of Transformation, by Michael Pollan.

I cook a lot, and I cook very well, thank you, and as a result I eat wonderfully. The recipes in this book are both my own creations and adaptations. They aren't complicated or fussy. They are what I enjoy and thrive on. I hope you enjoy them as well.

And now, let me explain who the Cooking Ape is. I am the Cooking Ape, and so are you. Cooking set our ancestors on the evolutionary path to humanhood. Cooking made food more digestible, and provided us with more nutrition in less time. That abundant nutrition fed a big, growing brain, while the shorter eating periods (chewing raw food takes an enormous amount of time) freed us to pursue other activities.

Cooking allowed us to grow socially. We learned cooperation and sharing. We learned to coordinate as a group, which allowed us to expand and flourish.

Cooking also made us the handsome creatures we are today. The less demanding requirements of eating cooked food changed our physiques. Our jaws and teeth got smaller. Even our lips thinned and became less muscular, because we didn't need them to crush raw food against our teeth anymore.

Our tums got smaller because we didn't need to consume and inefficiently digest large quantities of tough, raw food.

So smile when you stand before the mirror. You are seeing the reflection of a good-looking cooking ape, and thank goodness for that!

For a more extensive explanation of the influence cooking has had on us, read CATCHING FIRE, How Cooking Made Us Human, by Richard Wrangham. He may have been one of the first people to nickname us, 'The Cooking Ape'.

And finally, who is the <u>Healthy</u> Cooking Ape? I am, and with the Defiant Diet, you can be one, too.

A WORD ON FERMENTED FOODS (2)

We are the Cooking Apes. We are also the Fermenting Apes, because fermenting is a form of cooking.

Think about it. Fermenting, like other cooking, pre-digests our food, making it easier for our bodies to process.

Fermenting has many benefits for us. It is a way to preserve our food, which freed up considerable time for our ancestors to develop crucial talents and capabilities, and to become us.

Fermenting is also very, very healthy, providing our guts with a living culture of beneficial bacteria. These bacteria are probiotic (as opposed to antibiotic). They help our bowels absorb nutrition, and they help our bodies avoid/fight illness.

Let's not forget that fermentation also produces wine and beer!

For an extensive explanation on this subject, visit Sandor Katz's site: wildfermentation.com. Sandor is an extraordinary expert on fermentation, and is a joy to read. He is *the* source for info on this subject. I highly recommend learning from him.

I've embraced a handful of fermentation recipes, and always have the following in my 'fridge:

Brined cucumber slices

Crème fraiche (which is similar to sour cream, but better)

Brined shredded cabbage

And, infrequently, improved cultured buttermilk.

A word on brining: Brining requires salt, typically two tablespoons per quart of water. You make the call on whether this is a good choice for you personally. I'm not afraid, okay, *concerned* about salt. If you are, you can skip brining, BUT you'll be missing some delicious and otherwise beneficial food!

BRAISED SKIN-ON CHICKEN THIGHS (3)

Dark meat is where the flavor is. Chicken thighs are all dark meat. They are also easy and forgiving to cook. (For a funny, if coarse example of how forgiving they are, search Google for an editorial titled, How To Barbecue Chicken Thighs: A Guide For People Who Aren't Assholes).

Braising keeps the meat moist, and provides a wonderful sauce.

Make extra when you use this recipe. You'll appreciate the leftovers.

INGREDIENTS:

Skin-on chicken thighs

Diced onions

Thinly sliced celery

Thickly sliced carrots

Sage, thyme & any spices you feel go with poultry.

Salt & pepper

Olive oil

Chicken stock

½ - 1 cup of dry red wine

Sage leaves for garnish (not nec'y, but nice)

EQUIPMENT:

Oven proof pan that can also be used on the stove top. A stainless steel roasting pan works well here, as does a large stainless sauté pan. You don't want your pan to be too large, or you'll need too much stock, and the sauce flavor will be diluted.

PROCEDURE:

Prick the skin with a sharp knife, so the fat will render more efficiently when you are browning the thighs.

Season the thighs, including under the skin, with your choice of spices.

Brown the thighs on the stove top in a little olive oil. This can take 6-10 minutes for the skin side, and 3-4 minutes on the bald side. You may need to do this in more than one batch.

Set the thighs aside.

Drain most of the chicken fat from the pan…BUT SAVE IT!! This is my version of schmaltz, and it is delicious for cooking other foods. Store it in the 'fridge.

Bring the pan, with its browned bits stuck to the bottom, back to heat, and sauté the onions, celery and carrots for a few minutes.

Pour the red wine into the pan, and cook (with the veggies) for a few minutes to reduce and concentrate the flavors. Be sure to scrape all the brown bits off the pan bottom…they are tasty, tasty components of this dish.

Lay the chicken thighs on top of the vegetables, skin-side up.

Pour in enough chicken stock to come approximately ½ to 2/3 up the sides of the thighs.

Bring to light boil.

Lay 1 or 2 sage leaves on top of each chicken thigh.

Place pan in preheated 400 degree oven and cook for 30-45 minutes, until internal temp reaches the point you want.

Remove pan from oven, then remove thighs to a separate plate.

Heat the roasting pan and contents on the stovetop, bringing to a boil.

Cook for several minutes to reduce the stock a bit. This concentrates the flavor.

Return the chicken thighs to the pan, and cook a few minutes more to reheat them.

Plate the thighs and sauce and serve.

BREAD-LESS SANDWICHES (4)

Sorry, there really ain't no such thing. The definition of sandwich is, 'a filling between two slices of bread'.

Abandoning bread is probably the hardest aspect of going carb-free. It is worth it, but it is hard, especially when you can remember the taste of sandwiches, toast, buns, rolls, garlic bread, chiabatta bread, grilled bruschetta.....STOP!

I hesitate to tell you a truth; just as you'll remember the taste of a cigarette for twenty years after quitting smoking, you'll always remember the taste of forbidden carbs. Sorry.

There is an alternative. You needn't resort to eating sandwich fillings with a spoon, you can place the fillings in lettuce instead. Romaine is especially suited for use as a wrap, but you should experiment with bib lettuce, radicchio and other varieties.

Try it. You'll like it. You will.

QUICK BREAKFAST IDEAS (5)

Loosen up your concept of breakfast, and you'll greatly expand your choices. You've heard of people (maybe your own family) who get a kick out of having 'breakfast' food for dinner occasionally. Well, you can apply the same idea to what you eat in the morning, meaning have 'lunch' or 'dinner' food for breakfast.

However, many of us also want 'quick' food for breakfast. Okay. Leftovers from dinner are quick. But you know what is quicker? Let me give you a few ideas:

Cheese is marvelous for a quick breakfast. Have a slice or two of Havarti wrapped around some mild peppers or olive relish. How about a tablespoon (or two) of a nice blue cheese, with an accompaniment of walnuts? Cheddar with salted nuts? Cream cheese and pickles? Cottage cheese with halved cherry tomatoes and olive oil?

On the subject of cottage cheese, I'd like to again emphasize an important approach: read the ingredients on your food labels! You want the cleanest, least chemically influenced product on the grocery shelf. I've found Daisy cottage cheese to be the best.

Another quick food for breakfast is fresh fruit. I wouldn't go overboard here because of the natural sugar content, but a couple of ripe plums or a juicy peach in season, along with a bit of protein, will hold you very nicely. Apples are another simple item for your breakfast menu.

Eggs are a traditional breakfast food, but I reserve cooking them for the weekends. On work days I don't want to take the time to cook them, but that doesn't mean I forego eggs, especially since they are an incredibly beneficial food. I include them by hard-boiling several on the weekend, and storing them in an open container of water in the 'fridge.

Here is Julia Childs' technique for boiled eggs: Prick broad end of eggs, to allow expanding gas to escape during boiling without cracking the shell. Place eggs in a pan with enough cold water to cover them by an inch. Bring to a boil, cover, turn off heat, and leave for 17 minutes, then remove to an ice bath for two minutes, then return to boiling water for 10 seconds, and, cracking them against the edge of the sink, return the eggs to ice water bath.

The boiling water/ice water/boiling water/ice water sequence helps separate the shell from the egg, and makes peeling easier.

All right, now peel the eggs under running water and store, as described above.

Preparing and storing eggs like this turns them into convenience food. For example, you can make a batch of deviled eggs one evening (a very quick job), cover them with plastic wrap, and they are waiting for you the next morning…homemade breakfast fast food.

These stored eggs are also a great source of protein at other meals. Think egg salad, sliced eggs on greens, etc.

Meats can be another quick part of your breakfast. Nuke pre-cooked bacon or pancetta. Wrap ham slices around something savory. Or, if you have a little extra time, re-heat some leftover steak (yes, it is possible to have left-over steak, especially if you do it purposely) in a frying pan with a fried egg…gad is *that* good!

Cold cooked chicken is quick and tasty.

Try a forkful of smoked salmon.

Finally, don't forget avocados…one of nature's fast foods.

BRINED CUCUMBER SLICES (6)

This is the simplest pickle recipe I have used. It produces an excellent treat to nibble on while you are taking in live culture. Interestingly, the brine is as beneficial as the cuke slices, and can be sipped as a healthy elixir after fermentation.

INGREDIENTS:

Pickle-sized cucumbers. The quantity depends on you.

Fresh dill weed.

Sea salt. Two tablespoons per quart of water. Finely ground sea salt is easier to dissolve.

Water

PROCEDURE

Wash and slice the cukes into coins of your preferred thickness. I like about ½ inch.

Place the cuke coins in jar(s), layering with plenty of fresh dill.

Cover cukes with brine at a ratio of two tablespoons of sea salt per quart of water.

(When making the brine, I pour a few cups of boiling water over the salt in a large mixing bowl, to dissolve it, and then add ice water to bring the temperature down.)

Cap the jar(s) firmly and leave at room temperature for three days.

(I place the jars in an old cooler because they can leak as fermentation releases gas. The cooler will also contain any debris, should the jars explode. I have never, ever had this problem, but it pays to be careful…)

Inspect the jars during the three day waiting period. Twist them a little, and you should see bubbles climbing toward the top. This is good!

After three days, open the jars over a sink. They should bubble or even fizz…that's what you want, because it indicates fermentation.

Refrigerate the jars to stop the fermentation. Enjoy. Yum!

CANOLA OIL AND SNEAKY HEALTH SURPRISES (7)

Just a quick note here on the wisdom of questioning foods and ingredients. It is common knowledge that many of the items we grew up trusting are not worthy of that trust. Take margarine, for example. How about refined flour and white bread?

Well, to make my point, here's another one: canola oil. The 'healthy' aura that this oil has been wrapped in is…questionable! Do you know what canola stands for? Can (for Canadian), O (for oil), L (for low) and A (for acid). Yep. See, the marketers thought that canola oil sounded better than rapeseed oil. Google this baby to learn more. It is disturbing.

In fact, there is extensive research that warns against consuming many processed seed oils, including soybean, sunflower, canola, cottonseed, soybean, safflower, and other oil of this type.

On the other hand, olive oil and coconut oil are very healthy. Personally, I include butter as a healthy cooking fat. For high heat I use avocado oil.

So, be skeptical. Research what you are sticking in your mouth. We'll never be perfect in our food awareness, but the more curious we are, the healthier we'll be.

CARB-FREE BLT'S (8)

A home grown tomato sitting on the windowsill beckons like a scarlet siren, singing alluringly of salads and sauces, and…BLT's!

Rejoice, my carb-free friend. You may have BLT's without carbs. Just don't use bread. Think about it. BLT stands for Bacon, Lettuce & Tomato. There is no mention of bread in this acronym.

Here is what you do: Cut your luscious tomatoes into chunks, and place in a large bowl. Add mayo (I like Kewpie mayo, available at Walmart) and cooked, chopped bacon. Add salt and pepper, mix and serve with a side of radicchio or romaine leaves for scoops/wraps.

Is this as good as BLT's on good, toasted bread?

C'mon, why ask that question?

CHICK UNDER BRICK (9)

This cooking method uses foil wrapped brick(s) to press chicken pieces down firmly during the second phase of frying, when the pieces are skin-side down. The goal is to produce the best browning/crisping possible.

I used this technique years ago with chicken pieces, then forgot about it until I watched Jacques Pépin cook this way. He explained that Cornish hens are similar to the birds he cooked in France. What he did looked good, so I tried it. I enjoyed the Cornish hens, but more importantly, Michele was enthused about the dish, and asked when we would have it again. That is high praise, believe me.

INGREDIENTS:

2 Cornish hens.

Spices of choice, such as salt & pepper, cayenne pepper, cumin, sage, thyme, etc.

Oil for frying…you know I like avocado oil for frying.

EQUIPMENT:

A frying pan, preferably stainless steel, that is large enough to accommodate 2 split Cornish hens (4 halves).

Two aluminum foil wrapped bricks. As an alternative, you can use a heavy, weighted pan for pressing on the hens, but I don't think that is the best choice.

A thin-bladed fish turning spatula is handy for separating the hens from the pan in the end. The pieces tend to stick, which is fine, because you want those browned bits.

PROCEDURE:

Split the hens, using a large, heavy knife, or a cleaver.

Cut the spine from the ribs, and discard.

Spice both sides of the pieces generously.

Fry bone side down for 8-10 minutes.

Turn skin-side down, top with the bricks, positioning them to press all pieces downward, and cook for approx. 20 minutes.

Check for doneness with a thermometer, or by piercing.

Pry the pieces out of the pan, set aside.

Drain off and discard the fat in the pan, then deglaze the pan, while on heat, with a little white wine, chicken stock or water, scrubbing the pan's bottom with a wooden spatula to release the flavorful bits.

Pour the simple sauce over the split hens, serve and enjoy.

COFFEE BREAK BROTH (10)

Before leaving the house on business days, I throw together a thermos of Coffee Break Broth, which I later enjoy midmorning at the office. It is good tasting, healthy, and sustaining, and I look forward to filling my coffee mug with it at break time.

My ingredients may seem atypically numerous to you. Not to worry. This is a dish that cries out for your customization. Eliminate or substitute ingredients as you prefer. Your version needs to be tasty to YOU, and it needs to be convenient for YOU to make.

You'll notice that I include olives. I love olives. For cooking, I especially like oil-cured olives. They are wonderful in omelets, on pizzas (for my wife, since I don't eat carbs anymore), in veggie sautées and in my broth.

I keep a container of toothpicks in my desk drawer, and use one each day to spear the olives that remain at the bottom of my mug after I drink the liquid. The oil-cured olives have dark pits, and I expect that the cleaning crew thought a goat had crapped in my waste basket when I started eating this broth at the office.

You'll also notice that I include coconut oil. This is more a health choice than a taste choice (although the taste is pleasant). I do believe that coconut oil is good for you, but it is not a necessary ingredient. You might do a little research on your own, to help you decide whether you want to use coconut oil.

Combine the following ingredients (or your modified version) in a sauce pan and bring just to the boil, then transfer to your thermos. It is a good idea to pre-warm your thermos with hot water.

FLEXIBLE INGREDIENT LIST:

Organic broth/stock per thermos capacity. I use organic chicken stock from Costco.

Your choice of two types of olives…maybe six+ of each.

Heavy dash of turmeric (healthy choice and flavor).

Light dash of cumin (health and flavor).

Heavy sprinkle of dried dill.

Dash of celery salt.

Scattering of black pepper

Salt ONLY if you don't include olives.

Heaping tablespoon of coconut oil (see description above).

CREAMY DILLED CUCUMBER SLICES (11)

These cuke slices, like olives, try my self-control.

1-3 cukes

Large onion

Crème fraiche (or sour cream)

Rice vinegar or white vinegar

Fresh or dried dill

Kosher salt or sea salt

Black pepper

Optional: Large onion sliced and halved

Slice cukes into 1/8" thick coins, either with a knife or with a mandolin (watch those fingers!). Layer coins in a colander in the sink, sprinkling each layer with salt. This step draws moisture out of the coins. Leave colander in sink for ½ hour, then rinse the cuke slices thoroughly.

Meanwhile, if using: Slice the onion into thin rings, then cut the rings in half and separate. You may rinse the onion pieces under cold water if you want to reduce their pungency.

Pour enough crème fraiche or sour cream into a large bowl to eventually cover the cuke slices. Add enough vinegar to achieve a thick-soup texture. Add plenty of dill and pepper. Be careful with the salt…you may not need any more because of the residual salt in the slices.

Add the cuke coins and onions to the mixture, stir and refrigerate.

You can eat them immediately, but the cuke slices get better and better the longer you leave them. Don't be alarmed if froth develops; it is friendly bacteria improving the taste for you.

CRÈME FRAICHE (It's better than sour cream) (12)

Crème fraiche is similar to sour cream, but is better tasting, and making it yourself results in a much cleaner product. Making it yourself is also incredibly less expensive than buying the dinky, high priced jars at the deli.

Making crème fraiche is literally as simple as mixing two ingredients together and walking away.

You'll use it everywhere you would use sour cream, plus you can add it to sauces and other cooked dishes because it takes heat well without 'breaking'.

You can use it over berries or tomatoes.

You can make terrific dilled cucumber slices with it.

Crème fraiche is the result of the bacterial culture in the buttermilk fermenting the heavy cream.

One benefit of eating homemade crème fraiche is that you will be ingesting live culture, which is good for your innards.

INGREDIENTS:

One part store-bought cultured buttermilk (or one part previously made crème fresh)

Four parts heavy (whipping) cream. I buy it by the half gallon at Costco.

PROCEDURE:

Some recipes call for heating the heavy cream to 100 degrees. I stopped doing that, and it hasn't made a difference. I like to keep things simple.

Pour one part butter milk and four parts heavy cream into a clean jar. I find quart jars to be most manageable. A half-gallon of heavy cream and a pint of buttermilk will make almost three quarts of crème fraiche.

Stir briefly to combine.

Place the open jars on the counter and cover with a cloth. A dark cloth or tea towel is preferable.

Check after one day. If there is separation, stir to make sure the ingredients are well-blended. You want to make sure that the culture from the buttermilk is distributed evenly throughout the heavy cream.

Continue to check every day or two, stirring as necessary.

The crème fraiche should be as firm as sour cream by the fourth or fifth day. If it isn't, leave it for another day or two.

Cap and refrigerate the jars once you have reached the desired firmness. It will keep for at least a month.

FORAGING IN THE 'FRIDGE (13)

Following are examples of cooking a meal with what you have on hand.

I often start with onions. They are, after all, one critical leg in the 'holy trinity' of some cooking cultures, with celery and bell pepper (or carrots) often being the other legs. There are scientific reasons for these choices, including the presence of umami. The French, whose cooking techniques were developed over centuries, and became the code of Western cuisine, knew what they were doing.

Anyway, this weekend I diced and slowly sautéed a few yellow onions in butter. Then I added diced green bell pepper. Then I added julienned carrots.

Meanwhile, in a separate pan, I started brats in ½ inch of water, then after 10-15 minutes, when the liquid was gone, I sautéed the brats in a little olive oil until they were browned.

Then I removed the brats and slid a few cups of freshly cut tomatoes into the brat pan. The tomatoes released juice immediately, which deglazed the delicious browned bits from the bottom of the pan and gave the developing dish a much deeper flavor.

I also threw in some leftover cooked green beans and roasted tomatoes.

You see my point; use what is on hand.

Finally, I combined the onions/peppers/carrots with the tomatoes, and asked my wife to taste for spicing. She has good taste. She suggested a little pepper.

Now it was time to serve, and now was when I made my mistake…I put the brats into the vegetable stew.

"What do you think?" I asked as we ate.

"You shouldn't have put the brats in at the end. They steal the brightness from the veggies. The veggies don't taste like they did when they were alone in their own pan. It's good, but not as good as it was before you made them into a muddle. Separate, but equal, darlin'."

Well, there you are. Some foods make good neighbors but poor roomies.

However…I redeemed myself the next night. This time I chose leftover deboned meat from a rotisserie chicken we'd had a few nights before. Tasty deboned chicken loves a sauce, especially a gravy. This I was sure (and I was right) was going to be a dish where combining would be beneficial.

Again with the onions. Fine dice. Sauté in butter. Add a few roasted tomatoes.

Gravy needs drippings. I didn't have any, so I diced a raw chicken breast and crisped the little pieces in olive oil in a separate pan. My intention was to produce tasty, stuck-on brown bits. I let the diced chicken cook undisturbed, browning wonderfully, then stirred a few times and let it brown again. I added a little spicing. Salt, pepper, poultry seasoning.

The browned chicken bits came out of the pan. I then deglazed the pan with a little white wine and cooked the wine down to almost dry, and then got ready to make…GRAVY!

(Gravy is something I hadn't attempted before, but I was motivated by two issues; jarred gravy isn't as clean as I prefer, and my daughter, who has Celiac disease, can't eat the commercial stuff.)

The challenge was to make tasty, gluten-free chicken gravy. I had Googled the subject previously, and had learned that King Arthur makes a gluten free flour. Yes, that's right. It has rice flour, etc.

My daughter read the label and okayed the flour.

So here we go. Add 2-3 tablespoons butter to the hot, deglazed chicken pan, then add a similar amount of flour, and whisk for at least a couple of minutes over heat to make a roux. You must heat and stir for a few minutes to cook the flour. Raw floor doesn't taste good.

(Okay, okay, this isn't 100% carb-free because of the flour, BUT it isn't a significant amount per serving.)

After a few minutes of whisking and cooking, start to add chicken stock. Keep adding stock and whisking until you have the consistency you want. All this time, the deglazed brown bits are flavoring the developing gravy.

Now for the kicker flavoring. I added the sautéed onions and roasted tomatoes, and the chewy diced chicken bits to the gravy. Oh, baby this was developing nicely.

Finally, the deboned chicken went into the gravy/sauce, and I simmered everything until warmed through.

"What do you think?" I asked as we ate.

"It tastes like gravy," my wife said, approvingly, then added, "next time, don't cut the chicken you used for browning into such small pieces. They're really chewy. Good flavor, but a little distracting."

Oh, boy.

FORTIFIED CULTURED BUTTERMILK (14)

Cultured buttermilk is a fermented food, and a source of live culture. I'm a strong supporter of live culture, and I sometimes include buttermilk in my diet, but I limit it. Buttermilk is one food that increases my weight. I love it, but…

I want *good* buttermilk when I do drink it. I want thick, luscious, tangy buttermilk like I had when I was a kid. (That would be over half a century ago.)

Store-bought buttermilk is made with lowfat milk, which cripples the cultures ability to produce the flavor and texture I prefer. I have found a solution: give the culture a better diet.

This recipe is as simple as crème fraiche, two ingredients, and the process is exactly the same.

Tip: Try sprinkling salt and pepper on your buttermilk before drinking. Seriously. That's how I learned to drink it, and it is delicious.

INGREDIENTS:

Two parts organic whole milk. DO NOT use skim or 2% or anything else!

One to two parts store bought cultured buttermilk.

PROCEDURE:

Mix the two components together and pour into jar(s).

Store open jars at room temp, covered by a cloth (tea towels are good).

The mixture will 'clabber' (read *thicken*) after a few days. You can let it go for five days, if you like.

Cap the jars and place in 'fridge when it reaches the state you prefer.

It will easily keep for a few weeks. Fermentation is a method of preservation, after all.

FRIED GREEN TOMATOES (15)

These are fantastic to eat for breakfast with easy-over eggs. The green tomato slices are spicy and delicious, and their acidity is an excellent counterpoint to the creamy egg yolks.

This recipe produces excellent results, unlike the crap I once had at a Longhorn Steakhouse, where it was a new item on the menu, and they botched the hell out of it.

 I found the following spice mix in an old Paul Prudhomme recipe book. The tempura-style batter is from a Jacques Pepin video I watched while serving time on the treadmill.

To be totally carb-less, you can cook these slices without batter, and they are good, but, honestly, the batter makes them a lot better. And it is a thin batter, if you must rationalize using it.

INGREDIENTS:

2-3 large, green tomatoes.

Seasoning mix (1 ¼ teaspoons black pepper, 1 teaspoon salt, ¾ teaspoon cayenne pepper, ½ teaspoon garlic powder).

¼ inch (or a bit less) of oil for frying. I have found that avocado oil is the very best oil for this type of frying.

THE BATTER:

Approx. ¾ cup all-purpose flour.

Approx. 1 teaspoon baking *powder*.

One egg yolk.

Enough cold club soda to make a thin batter.

PREP AND EXECUTION:

Slice the stem end and bottom off of the tomatoes (you want the meat of the tomato exposed on both sides of the slices).

Cut the tomatoes in ¼" slices, and place on a plate or cutting board.

Sprinkle the seasoning mix on both sides of the slices, pressing the mix into the flesh.

Let the slices rest for at least 15 minutes. You will notice seepage, which is good.

Heat the oil in the skillet.

While the oil is heating, mix the batter. This batter relies on a chemical reaction between the baking powder and the club soda, and must be mixed immediately before use. It doesn't keep.

For the batter, mix the dry ingredients (flour and baking *powder*) in a bowl, stir in the egg yolk and then add a little club soda. Beat vigorously to combine and eliminate lumps, then add enough additional club soda to make a thin, light batter. It should be almost soupy. You'll be impressed with the frothiness.

Dip the tomato slices into the batter, remove and allow to drip for a moment, then ease them into the hot oil and leave alone for 3-5 minutes. The oil should be gently bubbling. Turn and cook for another 3-5 minutes. Remove and drain on a wire rack, or on paper towels.

Enjoy. And it is okay to munch a little of the excess batter that has crisped up. You aren't going to cook this dish very often.

FRITTATA (16)

A frittata is made by combining beaten eggs with a variety of pre-cooked ingredients, and cooking until set. There is the stovetop method, and there is the oven method. I prefer the oven method, since the dish is heated from all sides, and not just from the bottom.

You may eat your frittata immediately, or refrigerate and eat within a day, either cold or reheated. Imagine sending slices of this to the office or to school in a chilled lunch box. Or take them to a picnic. Or use them as human fuel on a road trip.

You are going to start this dish on the stovetop, and then finish in the oven, so you will need an oven-proof pan. Cast iron is traditional. I prefer an oven-proof nonstick pan, both because it is lighter, and because it will always wash up easily. Yes, yes, I've heard about how a well-seasoned cast iron pan is like a nonstick pan, but I've had experiences where that wasn't quite true.

INGREDIENTS:

6-8 eggs (you will get a feel for how many eggs you personally need after cooking this dish once).

Any combination of veggies and meats you would consider using in an omelet, such as diced onions (always onions, of course), chopped sun-dried tomatoes, chopped bell pepper, cooked andchopped bacon, ground sausage, cubed ham, smoked salmon, pitted olives, chives, etc., etc.

Cheese of your choice for topping.

Butter & olive oil for sautéing.

Salt, pepper and any other spices you prefer. Maybe some smoked paprika or cayenne pepper?

PROCEDURE:

Sauté all ingredients, excepting eggs and cheese, until cooked.

Loosely beat the eggs, and pour into the pan.

Stir to combine, and step back.

Cook undisturbed on stovetop until edges begin to pull away.

Sprinkle cheese on top of the frittata, and put pan into 350 degree oven.

Cook until the eggs set. I would check at approx. 12 minutes.

Slide cooked frittata onto a plate or cutting board, slice and serve.

TIP: If the cooked frittata doesn't slide out of the pan easily, use the omelet-freeing method of whacking the pan sideways against the heel of your covered hand (the pan is hot!), jarring the frittata and encouraging it to move.

Sour cream or crème fraiche and salsa are pleasant toppings.

HIGH PROTEIN CLAM CHOWDER & OYSTER STEW (17)

Canned clam chowder is a departure from totally carb-free, because of the potatoes. Canned oyster stew doesn't have as many carbs, but, like chowder, has a plethora of unpronounceable ingredients. So don't eat these very often. (But they *are* wonderfully tasty.)

I enjoy both of these canned soups, and have found a few ways to increase the flavor and protein content. First, buy cans/tins of clams and oysters, then drain and add the meat to the appropriate soup (clam meat to chowder, oysters to stew). Next, use half & half rather than milk. Finally, add a generous amount of butter at the end of heating.

Tip: Drain the extra clams and oysters into a glass, and then enjoy the liquid.

Addl Tip: If you are a man, do not offer this liquid to your woman. Well, not unless you want that unwelcome, 'What is *wrong* with you?' look.

HOMEMADE LABNEH (yogurt "cheese") (18)

This recipe is ridiculously simple: add a little salt to plain yogurt and let it drain for a day or two. You'll produce a very firm yogurt "cheese" that will keep in the 'fridge for weeks. It has a texture approaching cream cheese, and a fuller flavor than the original yogurt.

I've read that in the Middle East this is used with added olive oil and spices as a dip. I use it as a quick bit of protein for breakfast. A heaping tablespoon of labneh and a raw plum, for example, are enough to see me happily to coffee break.

Note: the liquid that drains from the yogurt is called whey, and is a source of live, beneficial culture. I drink it.

INGREDIENTS:

Plain yogurt…the cleanest, with lowest sugar content you can find.*

A pinch of salt…preferably sea salt

EQUIPMENT:

2 Bunn type flat bottom paper coffee filters

Strainer

Bowl for mixing

Bowl for catching strained whey

PROCEDURE:

Mix a pinch of salt into your yogurt. Don't be over generous with the salt.

Line your strainer with one coffee filter.

Place your strainer on a bowl that is deep enough to accommodate the draining whey, while keeping the strainer out of the accumulating liquid.

Pour the salted yogurt into the strainer, and lay the other, flattened, coffee filter on top of the mixture.

Place the bowl and strainer into your 'fridge, and leave for at least a day. I think two days is better.

When the labneh has reached your preferred consistency, remove it from the strainer and coffee filters, and transfer it to a closable container and store it in the 'fridge. It is ready to use.

*By 'clean', I mean unadulterated, with no unhealthy or mysterious ingredients. Read the labels! And if you compare brands for sugar content, you'll find that Fage has less than Dannon or Yoplait.

IMPROVED OMELET TECHNIQUE (19)

This pointer is also covered in the Kitchen Tips section.

My omelet pan looks like a toy because it is only 8". My wife thought it was cute when it arrived from Amazon. Cute-schmoot! This baby is ideal for fried eggs, frittatas, scrambled eggs and of course, omelets.

It is annoyingly difficult to find a decent 8" nonstick omelet pan with a glass lid. As I mentioned, I found ours on Amazon. It is a Simply Calphalon Enamel 8" Covered Omelet Pan, and cost $30.

The lid is essential, especially for turning omelets (see following technique).

Omelet Turning Technique Using Lid: Flipping omelets and frittatas freehand is iffy. Sometimes you are successful, and other times you look like a hack. You can get 100% positive results by using your lid to turn them. The classic technique, which I have improved on, is to cook the first side, then place a plate on the pan, quickly turn the pan upside down, which releases the food onto the plate, and then slide the upturned, sloppy mess back into the pan. Yuck! You get runny stuff all over your plate, which is not only messy, but wasteful.

My improved technique is to cook the first side, and then carefully tilt the pan and slide the omelet onto the overturned lid that you are holding in your other hand like a platter. At this point you are looking at the uncooked topside of the omelet or frittata, which is resting in the lid. Now you turn the empty pan upside down and fit it onto the upside down lid, whereupon you quickly turn the joined parts right-side-up, and you end up with the uncooked side on the bottom. Very, very neat and satisfying.

KITCHEN TIPS (20)

PANS:

OVENPROOF STAINLESS STEEL SAUTE PAN WITH LID

I have a four quart straight sided All-Clad sauté pan. It was pricey, $200+, but it is a magnificent pan. I use it more often than my nonstick. Don't be alarmed at this idea, thinking that clean-up would be a problem. Clean-up is actually very easy if you add water to the pan right after using, and leave it to soak while you eat your meal. The pan will wipe out quite nicely after you dine. You'll be surprised.

Clean-up is even easier if you deglaze the pan for a reduction sauce. It just about cleans itself.

A lid is important. There are times you'll want to steam a bit before continuing the sauté.

Ovenproof is also important. There are times you'll want to finish a dish in the oven after sautéing.

STAINLESS STEEL SAUCE PANS WITH GLASS LIDS

Heavy bottoms are a desirable feature in sauce pans, because they distribute the heat and reduce hot spots. Glass lids are also best, because they allow you to observe what is happening, without removing the lid and losing heat.

I like to have at least 2-3 sauce pans of various sizes. Quality is a must. You'll get over the sticker shock when you enjoy their practicality and longevity. These are pans you'll have for a lifetime.

NONSTICK OMELET PAN WITH GLASS LID

My omelet pan looks like a toy because it is only 8". My wife thought it was cute when it arrived from Amazon. Cute-schmoot! This baby is ideal for fried eggs, frittatas, scrambled eggs and of course, omelets.

It is annoyingly difficult to find a decent 8" nonstick omelet pan with a glass lid. As I mentioned, I found ours on Amazon. It is a Simply Calphalon Enamel 8" Covered Omelet Pan, and cost $30.

The lid is essential, especially for turning omelets (see following technique).

Omelet Turning Technique Using Lid: Flipping omelets and frittatas freehand is iffy. Sometimes you are successful, and other times you look like a hack. You can get 100% positive results by using your lid to turn them. The classic technique, which I have improved on, is to cook the first side, then place a plate on the pan, quickly turn the pan upside down, which releases the food onto the plate, and then slide the upturned, sloppy mess back into the pan. Yuck! You get runny stuff all over your plate, which is not only messy, but wasteful.

My improved technique is to cook the first side, and then carefully tilt the pan and slide the omelet onto the overturned lid that you are holding in your other hand like a platter. At this point you are looking at the uncooked topside of the omelet or frittata, which is resting in the lid. Now you turn the empty pan upside down and fit it onto the upside down lid, whereupon you quickly turn the joined parts right-side-up, and you end up with the uncooked side on the bottom. Very, very neat and satisfying.

NONSTICK SKILLETS

Nonstick pans are extremely useful. They can also be rather temporary, from one year to several years, depending on their quality, so (as with any of your pans) it is less expensive to pay for quality. Quality is not only cheaper in the long term, it is also much more pleasant to use.

We own three nonstick pans. One is the eight inch omelet pan, another is an eleven inch fry pan with a heavy bottom, and the last nonstick is twelve-thirteen inches. We store them, nested, in the oven, with hot pads in between to prevent scratching.

We do regret not being more thoughtful when we bought the largest pan online. It is shaped too much like a wok, making the flat bottom unacceptably small for the pan's overall size. We now need to swallow hard and buy a more suitable pan.

DON'T use metal utensils in your nonstick pans, regardless of the manufacturer's claims. I use wooden utensils and nylon or silicone spatulas.

Some nonstick pans are oven-proof to 350 degrees or so. This can be a desirable trait, especially when making fritattas.

STAINLESS STOCK POTS

As always, go for quality here. It is better to have one good stock pot than three cheapies. The cheap pots will pit, and are too thin to distribute heat efficiently. Try to be logical when you choose the size of your stock pot(s). If you don't need a large pot, don't buy it. Bigger isn't better. Bigger takes more energy during cooking, and more of your personal energy when you lug its heavy butt, full of liquids, from here to there.

STAINLESS STEEL ROASTING/LASAGNA PAN

A normal size pan of this sort (17-19") is very good for roasting, but we've found that a smaller version (14") is also appreciated. The big guy is useful for holidays and family gatherings, but you will enjoy the ease of handling that the smaller pan affords when you are cooking for just a few people.

Quality is paramount, of course. Spend some time considering the handle configuration on these pans. Think about how comfortable and accessible the handles will be during use, especially considering you'll be using hot pads or oven mitts to handle them. Think also of how conveniently/efficiently they will store/stack in your cupboard.

RIMMED BAKING SHEETS

These are great for any number of uses, from baking to broiling to keeping your counter clean when you are grating cauliflower. You'll want at least a couple of these. The larger sizes are the most useful, but infrequently you might appreciate a smaller version. You'll find these at Costco and restaurant supply stores (as well as online, of course). They are not expensive.

UTENSILS & GADGETS:

KNIVES

This is a crazy broad subject, and it is subjective. Use the knives you prefer, and keep them sharp!

I have a substantial chef-type knife for cutting large items, like cabbage and squash and turkeys. I bought it at a restaurant supply store for under $20.

I have a couple of OXO Good Grips 4" Santoku knives for medium cutting and slicing. They are in the $12 range.

I have several Victorinox 3.25" paring knives, which are about $6 on Amazon.

I have a Chinese style slicing cleaver that probably cost me $15 at the local grocery store, years ago.

You will have noticed that I'm a cheap*** when it comes to knives. That's okay with me. I'm satisfied with this selection. I'm not experienced with the high end blades, so I don't covet them. This is given proof by my boring knife skills. I'm not flashy when I'm cutting/slicing/dicing. My movements are deliberate, and my first knife priority is to not cut myself.

I do spend a lot on my sharpening equipment. The latest and greatest is the European Smooth and Serrated Knife Sharpener from Hammacher Schlemmer, at $120. I know, I know. That is a lot to spend to keep your knives sharp, but goodness, this thing does a wonderful job. It sits nicely on your counter top. It takes very little counter space. It has two spring-loaded cross-arms with sharpening surfaces, and it only takes a few quick pulls to maintain your edges. I give each knife a few licks on this darling every time I use them.

Do buy a steel if you don't use a handy sharpener. It will keep your edges better between sharpenings. You may or may not know the purpose of a steel. This utensil doesn't actually sharpen…it straightens. That's right. The thin, sharp edge of your blades curl over as you use them. Pulling your blades across a steel straightens out those curled edges. Steels are for maintaining, not sharpening.

FISH TURNING SPATULA

This is a specialized utensil that you will use much more often than you'd expect. The blade is made of thin, strong steel, and is bent slightly. The thinness of the blade material, and the angle of the blade allow this spatula to slide nicely under delicate fish, sure, BUT it works very, very well for releasing other meats during sautéing. You'll be surprised.

SPATULAS FOR NONSTICK PANS

We've gone through many nonstick spatulas over the years. The complaints have been that they were too thick, too thin, too stiff, too flexible, and so on. The spatulas we settled on (with satisfaction) are OXO Good Grips Nylon Flexible Turners. We have four of them because we use them so much that one or two are always in the dishwasher. They are inexpensive.

SPIDER SKIMMER

This is something like a little basket with a long handle. You'll use it where you've used a slotted spoon in the past. It is handy for boiled eggs, boiled potatoes, elbow pasta, coarse debris while making stock, etc.

I like an all stainless steel spider. It is much easier to clean than the Asian version, which has a woven brass basket and a bamboo handle. I've used both, and have since discarded the bamboo job.

SKIMMER

A plain skimmer differs from a spider in that this skimmer is much flatter, and has much smaller holes. It is made for skimming scum off stocks and other liquid dishes during simmers.

A plain skimmer works well in other situations, often better than the spider. I use ours to lift lettuce out of an ice water bath, which makes the job much more comfortable than using my hands. The flatness and small holes in the skimmer make it preferable to a spider.

My skimmer is an All-Clad T108 Stainless Steel Skimmer. It was $22 on Amazon.

TONGS

Regular old straight spring-loaded tongs work best for us. Their usefulness is much more universal than scissor-type tongs, or bent-legged tongs. We have straight tongs, and store them, straddled on the side of a salt glazed crock nest to the stove.

Be careful with specialized tongs. For example, we owned a spring steel set of asparagus tongs. Its design incorporated gripping ridges for securing the asparagus stalks. I suffered with that iffy utensil for some time, but it recently failed, once again, to grip as I tried to transfer stalks from the platter to my plate. It made a mini-mess on the tablecloth, and I threw the aggravating device into the recycle bin…with prejudice. I will not abide a tool or device that disappoints.

WIDE MOUTH FUNNEL

Wide mouth funnels are familiar to home canners. They are made of stainless steel, and rest securely on the top of wide mouth jars. They take the sloppiness out of pouring, especially when you are pouring from large vessels.

STAYBOWLIZER (AND DOUBLE-BOILER)

The first time you use a Staybowlizer you will marvel. It is simple, practical, and a wonderful solution for various situations. A Staybowlizer is a silicone ring/collar, that acts like a third hand when you are whipping liquids in bowls. You place the Staybowlizer on your counter, set your bowl into it, and you don't need to touch the bowl again until you are finished mixing. The sticky silicone secures the bowl in place while you whisk and whip. This is especially appreciated when you are drizzling oil with one hand, while beating with the other, as in vinaigrettes and homemade mayo.

The Staybowlizer also facilitates double boiling, because you can set it on the rim of a boiling pan, and then set a bowl into the tapered mouth on the collar. The silicone seals around pan top and the bowl bottom, and converts any number of pan/bowl combos into efficient double boilers. Very neat.

You can buy these babies on Amazon for about $20.

We store ours in the cupboard, under our stainless utility bowls.

EGG SLICER

Okay, this isn't a necessity. It does have its uses. It quickly and precisely slices hardboiled eggs. It does this job much better than your or I can with a knife.

Jacques Pepin does a cute trick with his egg slicer. He slices once, then turns the egg ninety degrees and slices again. This immediately creates rough-chopped egg salad.

The egg slicer can also slice strawberries efficiently.

I really like mine.

A KitchenAid egg slicer cost about $7 on Amazon, or you can find them at Bed Bath & Beyond.

STAINLESS STEEL VEGETABLE STEAMER BASKET

We prefer the butterfly type of steamer basket. It has perforated, hinged, overlapping 'petals' that adjust to your various sauce pan sizes. It is inexpensive, useful and durable.

PARCHMENT PAPER

If you haven't cooked with parchment paper, you are in for a pleasant surprise. I use it to line pans when I am roasting tomatoes, since I don't want tomatoes in contact with aluminum foil. I also use it for roasting other veggies. It makes clean-up much, much easier (I still feel trauma regarding scrubbing baking sheets, a mental injury that goes back to the summer I was a kitchen boy in a girls' camp).

Another wonderful use is the *en papillote* (in parchment) cooking method, where you make a pouch with parchment paper. You place your protein in the pouch with spices and sprigs of herbs, and a bit of olive oil or butter, and then seal the pouch and bake it. This works especially well for fish.

Cook with paper? Won't it catch on fire? Nope. Parchment paper can go up to 420 degrees. I've cooked with it at higher temps.

My favorite product in this category is Reynolds Smart Grid Parchment Paper, which has a grid, obviously, printed on the paper and comes on a roll, like wax paper. The grid is greatly appreciated when you need to cut a sheet of the paper to fit a pan.

A tip: Parchment paper retains its rolled attitude after you tear it off the mother roll. You can straighten the torn sheet by orienting it rolled side up, and then pulling it, diagonally, downward over the edge of a sharp counter edge, while maintaining tension. Repeat this from the opposing corner, and you'll have a very manageable, flat sheet of paper.

A great source of info and parchment paper products is www.paperchef.com.

STAINLESS STEEL COOLING/ROASTING RACK

I bought some of these racks years ago, pre-Defiant Diet, when I was trying to learn how to bake cookies, of all things. I've been off carbs and sugar for so long now that the idea of sweet foods is repulsive…really, it's true.

Now I use these racks for cooking meats in the oven. They allow the heat to surround the meat, and they allow the fat to drip off. Place the rack on a cookie sheet that is lined with aluminum foil or parchment paper. The lining facilitates clean-up.

I also use the racks out of the oven, for draining and resting fried foods.

Racks with a grid pattern are more useful. They prevent smaller items from slipping through.

MANDOLIN

There is one useful kitchen device that makes me nervous (and I used to be a machinist). That device is the mandolin, which is a simple concept, having an adjustable and *very sharp* blade in its bed, that slices food efficiently as you push the food item along the bed. You can slice cukes and carrots and celery and onions and your freaking finger tips if you aren't careful! The memory of slicing off a finger tip stays with you. Believe me.

Most mandolins do come with some sort of pushing device, but the things aren't always suitable, so you must then push with your unprotected hand. A mandolin's speed and efficiency can be painfully surprising. The critical safety measure you must follow *without fail*, is to keep your mind on the task, and stop a few snicks short of your tender digits. This safety measure is self-enforcing if you let your mind wander.

I am glad I have a mandolin. I use it frequently. And I respect the heck out of it.

PAN-SEARED STEAK (21)

Prepare to be converted to a new steak cooking technique: steak that is seared on the stove top and finished in the oven. You must try it to believe it. You may even turn your back on grilling steak after this experience.

First, I'll start with an obvious point, which is that you must use high quality meat. And it must be thick, at least 1 ½". I prefer well marbled, bone-in ribeye.

As a rare (pun acknowledged) treat, try organic, grass fed beef from a quality-conscious farmer sometime. This meat is so delicious that I even eat and relish the gristle. It is a rare treat because it costs twice as much as the steak we normally cook.

I sometimes buy a whole ribeye roast at Costco, and then cut it into steaks of the thickness I prefer.

The prep I use for steak is the same regardless of the cooking technique. I take the steak out of the 'fridge an hour before cooking, salt the be-jaysus out of it...no, no, I mean *really* salt it *heavily*...on both sides, and let it rest on a rack over a plate until just before cooking.

I pre-heat the oven to 450 degrees, and then preheat an oven-proof skillet (think All-Clad or cast iron) over medium to high heat on the stove top. I rinse the salt off the steak under cool water, pat it dry with paper towels, spread a thin film of olive oil on both sides, and drop it into the hot skillet. It must sizzle aggressively, because you want it to sear and form a tasty crust. This is why a thick steak is important. A thin steak would cook too quickly to develop that delicious crust.

Tip: cover the pan with a spatter guard.

You are going to sear the steak for a total of five minutes, four minutes on the first side, and one minute on the second side, then immediately put the pan into the preheated oven for another five minutes.

Remove the steak to a plate or platter, top with a patty of butter, tent with aluminum foil, and let rest for 5-10 minutes.

RESERVE the juices that are released during the resting period! Pour them over your portion of the steak, and you'll double the flavor!

Delicious. Wonderful crust from the sear. Moist, flavorful interior. Only salt and butter. Pure, healthy protein. Good fat for your brain. Probably fewer carcinogens than grilling.

To be kind, you should keep the cover on your outdoor grill while you are cooking this way, and swooning over the results...you don't want it to witness this joy through the patio door, or it will fear and fret for its future.

POWDERED CHEESE (22)

Powdered cheese?! Yep. No kidding. There truly is such a thing as powdered cheese. I really enjoy Cabot Powdered Cheddar, which is actually named Cabot Cheddar Shake!, because it is popular as a popcorn topping.

Okay, I accept that it must be tasty on popcorn, but that is not how I use it. I sprinkle it on scrambled eggs and omelets. I zing up steamed veggies with it. I use it in/on soups and salads. You should absolutely try it if you like cheese.

Bon Appétit has a crazy recipe (this is where I learned about Cabot's) using Cabot-sprinkled fried pork rinds as a base, with onions and guacamole and other vegetables for a chipless Mexican dish. It's pretty good.

You can google Cabot Cheddar Shake! to find Cabot's home page, which has a Where To Buy button. Be aware that while the suggested locations carry Cabot products, they might not carry the Cheddar Shake.

I buy mine online from Dakin Farm.

RED CABBAGE SLAW (23)

This is a general recipe, and welcomes your customization.

One head red cabbage, shredded.

½ red onion, sliced, separated and rinsed.

6 chopped green onions.

Mayo (I like the Kewpie brand).

A healthy glug of unpasteurized apple cider vinegar.

Salt & pepper.

Dried dill.

Celery salt.

Dried parsley, if fresh isn't available.

REDUCING ONION BREATH (24)

I have eaten raw onions for as long as I can remember. Unfortunately, it was half a century before I learned how to reduce and almost eliminate the resulting bad breath.

The fact that I've been happily married for 45 years is a mystery I choose not to explore here.

Here is the trick: Rinse the cut onion pieces under cold water.

It is that simple. Rinsing removes some of the sulfurous compounds that cause onion breath.

Don't over-rinse, or you'll get rid of the flavor as well. Just put the onion pieces in a sieve or colander, and give them a quick shower.

And that, my friend, is how you can avoid the unsettling, intimate, wifely question…."What have you been eating?"

ROASTED BELL PEPPERS (25)

Roasted bell peppers can be served as a warm side dish, or used on sandwiches, in salads, in omelets and as an ingredient in sautés. The recipe is simple and has a surprising ingredient: anchovies. Wait, wait, wait…you'll like these peppers. Even my wife likes them, and that says a lot.

INGREDIENTS:

5 assorted bell peppers

Coarsely chopped or sliced garlic

Anchovy fillets

Olive oil

Salt & Pepper

PROCEDURE:

Quarter the bell peppers at the seams, and remove the white pith.

Toss the pepper pieces in a little olive oil, and place, inside up, on a parchment lined cookie sheet. They will look like little canoes, waiting to cradle the following ingredients.

Drop a few pieces of garlic onto each piece of pepper.

Lay ½ anchovy fillet on each piece of pepper.

Lightly sprinkle with salt (the anchovies are already very salty)

Generously sprinkle with pepper

Put cookie sheet into 450 degree pre-heated oven for 30 minutes.

Use tongs to remove garlic and anchovies from the pieces after cooking.

ROASTED TOMATOES (26)

I roast ripe whole cherry tomatoes, sliced ripe large tomatoes, halved and seeded Roma tomatoes and even sliced green tomatoes. Roasting intensifies their flavor. You'll pull these out of the 'fridge to enhance any number of dishes. They are great on salads, pizzas, in omelets and as a snack.

My adult daughter packs quantities of these (ours) for her lunch. This practice has caused me moments of surprise and loss as I vainly searched the vegetable drawer in the refrigerator for roasted tomatoes that were there no more.

IMPORTANT: You should prick cherry tomatoes with a sharp knife to prevent them from bursting while roasting. You should also prick the skin of halved Roma's, to allow the moisture to cook away.

INGREDIENTS:

Cherry tomatoes, halved Romas or sliced large tomatoes

Olive oil

Salt & Pepper & various spices/herbs

PROCEDURE:

Line a cookie sheet with parchment paper.

Lay tomatoes on cookie sheet, skin-side down if using halved Romas.

Drizzle with olive oil.

Sprinkle with salt and pepper, dried oregano, etc.

Roast in 400 degree oven until the tomatoes collapse, with a few developing singed edges. This can take an hour or more…or less.

SALAD TIPS (27)

Salads are a big part of my diet. I'm not talking light foo-foo salads. I'm talking about full flavored, clean and satisfying salads.

I rarely use store-bought dressings (although I will *very* infrequently succumb to a bottle of seductive blue cheese dressing), instead opting for tasty extra virgin olive oil and a pleasant vinegar.

Now and then I'll make a container of simple vinaigrette. Oxo makes a dandy salad dressing shaker in two sizes, and they work well. You start with a few glugs of vinegar (enough to end with an approx. ratio of 1 part vinegar to 4 parts oil), add a tablespoon or so of Dijon mustard, toss in a minced shallot or some finely diced onion, sprinkle in salt and pepper, and then shake to combine. The mustard is important because it is an emulsifier, meaning that it helps the vinegar and oil to combine.

Once you have the initial ingredients shaken, it is time to add your oil in small increments. A little oil and shake. A little oil and shake. Taste near the end of the process and adjust the vinegar or oil as necessary.

Tip: Take the shaker of dressing out of the 'fridge before prepping your salad, to give it time to warm a little and become more pourable. If you forget to do this beforehand, you can set the chilled shaker in a bowl of warm water to reduce the dressings viscosity.

If you don't have a salad dressing shaker, make your dressing the old fashioned way by putting the vinegar and Dijon and spicing in a bowl, and then whisk constantly as you drizzle in olive oil.

Here is a tip for reducing the amount of olive oil you use in your salad: Place naked lettuce in a bowl and drizzle a teaspoon of olive oil over it, then mix gentle with your fingers. You'll be surprised at how little oil is needed to coat every piece of lettuce.

Here is a BIG tip: Use an ice-water bath to clean your lettuces. The cold water 'shocks' the leaves, rehydrates them, makes them crisper and extends their life by days. Both my wife and I were startled repeatedly when we first tried this washing method, because it kept the lettuce in great condition for five or six days.

To wash lettuce using the ice-water method, you simply get a large bowl and fill it half-way with water and a few cups of ice cubes. Put the chopped/cut/torn lettuce into the ice-water, swish it very gently, and leave for 5-10 minutes, then remove to a salad spinner basket, drain and spin. DO NOT *pour* the salad into the basket, or you'll be giving it a dirt shower! You must *lift* the lettuce out of the water, leaving the debris behind. This little procedure will save you money and reduce waste.

SOFT HARD-BOILED EGGS (28)

Some people drop 'hard' from the name and call these just soft-boiled eggs. Regardless of the name, they are simply eggs that have been boiled to the point where the white is fully set, and the yolk is not fully set. You can adjust the cooking time to achieve the yolk of your choice. The timing in this procedure makes for yolks that are very soft and creamy, but not liquid.

I once conducted a small and unscientific survey, which concluded that roughly half the local population loves soft-boiled eggs, while the remaining, stunted population shudders at the mention of less than concrete yolks (does that make them yoke-uls?).

The following method for soft hard-boiled eggs works beautifully, and the eggs peel with uniform ease (no small accomplishment). Two of my guiding lights, Julia Child and Jacques Pepin, have their own methods. I prefer Jacques' method for cooking, and Julia's for storage.

I use jumbo eggs.

1) Pierce the large end of the eggs with a push pin, or something similar, to allow the trapped air to escape during heating. There are inexpensive devices called (what else) Egg Piercers. You may want to buy one if you like boiled eggs.
2) Lower the eggs into enough boiling water to cover them and cook at a very gentle boil for 10 minutes.

   The low heat is necessary to prevent the chemical reaction that creates both a sulfurous odor and unattractive discoloration.

3) IMPORTANT! Drain off the water and shake the pan to crackle the eggshells. Don't go crazy here, or you'll split the eggs. I know this from experience.
4) Immediately put the eggs into an ice water bath, and leave for at least 15 minutes.
5) Peel under running water.
6) Store, covered with water, in an open container in the 'fridge.

STUFFED & BAKED ACORN SQUASH (29)

This was a frequent dish when I was a kid, but then, so was Finnan Haddie, which is smoked haddock baked in milk…but I digress.

My point is that some very nice, once common dinners, have been forgotten. They have gone the way of fish on Friday, which is a very sad loss, because that custom created demand, and that demand caused competition, and that competition resulted in excellent fish dining, both at home and at restaurants. Sigh.

That concludes my sermon.

Now onto delicious stuffed acorn squash. Don't be put off by the length of these ingredients and steps. This is really a very simple recipe, and you'll repeat it easily. I've learned to make it even easier by cooking the stuffing the previous day.

INGREDIENTS:

One acorn squash per two people.

Enough ground pork to fill squash hollows.

Diced onions.

Grated/shredded cooking apple. We feel this is a *very* important ingredient, because it complements the pork.

Salt & Pepper.

Sage.

Thyme.

Cooked, crumbled bacon (optional).

Grated cheese of choice.

Cinnamon*.

Maple syrup.

Butter and olive oil for sautéing.

PROCEDURE FOR SQUASH:

Split the acorn squash from stem end to bottom end, remove seeds and scrape cavity clean.

Place the squash halves in a glass baking dish, cut side down, and add ¼" of water.

Bake in a 375 degree oven for 30 minutes, then test for doneness by piercing with a sharp paring knife. Continue to bake until tender.

PROCEDURE FOR STUFFING (this may be cooked a day before):

Sauté onions and grated/shredded apple in butter and olive oil until soft.

Pull raw ground pork into small pieces, and add to sauté pan, then cook until browned.

Add crumbled bacon, if using.

Drizzle a little Maple syrup into the mix.

Add salt & pepper, sage and thyme to your taste.

Cook briefly to warm all ingredients, tasting and adjusting as nec'y.

FINALE:

Drain the water from the glass baking dish.

Turn acorn squash halves cut side up in the pan.

Rub a little butter on the squashes interiors, if you like.

Sprinkle the interior of the squash halves with cinnamon.*

Mound the ground pork mixture into the squash cavities and drizzle with Maple syrup.

Sprinkle grated cheese on top of the stuffing.

Return glass baking dish to oven and bake until brought up to heat and the cheese is melted.

*A NOTE ON CINNAMON: There is a good cinnamon (Ceylon), and there is a bad cinnamon (cassia or Chinese). You, like most of us, have almost certainly been eating the bad cinnamon. Cassia/Chinese cinnamon contains a high level of a dangerous substance. Ceylon cinnamon has a minute amount of that substance, and is much more flavorful. Unfortunately, Ceylon cinnamon is difficult, if not impossible, to find locally. One online source is Dru Era.

TACO SALAD WITH HOMEMADE TACO SEASONING (30)

For the Defiant Diet, you can certainly eat tacos (who doesn't love tacos?), as long as you forego the shells. This is not that difficult to do. Have a taco salad instead. You'll like it. You'll like it a lot.

For my serving of this salad I lay down a base of good lettuces on a large dinner plate, then add tomatoes, sliced olives, jalapeno slices and other veggies, drizzle with olive oil and a little vinegar, followed by salt and pepper. Then I sprinkle on a generous amount of shredded cheese. Then I plop on a nice portion of taco meat, topped with a generous amount of crème fraiche or sour cream. I finish this growing mound with a handful of diced onion, salsa and a couple of tablespoons of sambal oelek (a wonderful chili paste with a manageable amount of heat).

When your family looks disapprovingly at the quantity of material on your plate, you should indignantly reply, "It's mostly vegetables!"

You can use commercial taco seasoning for the ground beef, of course, but it isn't as 'clean' as making the mixture yourself. You'll see what I mean when you read the ingredients on the prepackaged stuff.

Homemade taco seasoning recipes tend to share universal ingredients. You can vary the ratios for your own taste. I seriously suggest making enough for a month, which for us means enough for at least four batches. See, our house has Taco Tuesday each week. You'll use two tablespoons of this seasoning per pound of ground beef. Store it in an airtight container.

INGREDIENTS FOR TACO SEASONING:

1 tablespoon chili powder

¼ tsp garlic powder

¼ tsp onion powder

¼ tsp crush red pepper flakes

½ tsp dried oregano

½ tsp paprika

1 ½ tsps. ground cumin

1 tsp sea salt

1 tsp black pepper

PROCEDURE FOR COOKING TACO MEAT:

Brown your ground beef.

Drain the resulting fat.

Stir in two tablespoons of the taco seasoning per pound of ground beef.

Add ¾ to 1 cup of water to the pan.

Stir, and simmer to allow meat to absorb the moisture.

Stand back and let the mob build its tacos and salads.

VEGGIE PASTA WITH CLAM SAUCE (31)

I became fascinated with 'spiralizing' squashes, carrots and other solid vegetables, after seeing a gadget ad on the internet. The gadget cut veggies into pasta-like strands. The strands were then used in salads (raw) and pasta dishes (slightly cooked). So, being a sucker for gadgets, especially cooking gadgets, I bought one of the advertised hourglass-shaped spiralizers.

The stupid thing broke the first time...*the first time*...I used it!

Nuts.

I was still intrigued with the idea, if dismayed by the device. Sure, I could try to produce pasta-like strands with my knives, but who the heck wants to spend that much time producing inconsistent results?

The little bulldog in my brain kept gnawing on this bone. I went to Bed, Bath & Beyond, and found an inexpensive solution. It is a dual-purpose mandolin; the Zyliss 2 in 1 Hand Held Slicer, which sells for $20.

This clever mandolin can produce coins of veggies, or, with the push of a button, can produce julienned, pasta-like strands. It is robust, inexpensive and satisfying to use. Google it.

(IMPORTANT: Be very, very careful when using the mandolin. Too many of us, myself included, had to learn the hard way. The mandolin slices very quickly, and your fingers can descend toward the blades faster than you realize. That is why a pusher comes with it.)

Meanwhile, I was reading about the history and science of cooking, and reacquainted myself with the concept of umami. Umami is the fifth taste sense, along with sweet, sour, bitter and salty. Umami is the Japanese word for 'deliciousness', and was identified in Japan in the early 1900's. You can Google this.

This fifth taste refers to savoriness, and is associated with glutamates. Umami makes the whole dish you are eating taste better. Mushrooms are one of the few foods high in umami. This gave me an idea: how about mincing mushrooms, then sautéing the be-Jayzus out of them, and using them as a base for a stew, soup, etc.?

I tried this idea, with very pleasant results. The directions follow. The mushrooms aren't critical to this dish, but they are most appreciated.

INGREDIENTS:

A few cups (at least) of finely minced regular white mushrooms.

Enough zucchini to produce a cup or two of strands per diner.

Enough summer squash for a cup or two per diner.

Canned/jarred clam sauce, either red or white.

Canned minced clams to fortify the clam sauce. (I often add additional protein to ready-made sauces and soups. I add minced clams to store-bought clam chowder, and canned oysters to store-bought oyster stew. More power, baby.)

Butter.

Olive oil.

Salt.

Beverage of choice.

PROCEDURE:

Mince the mushrooms. I mean *mince* the mushrooms. You can start mincing with a knife, but I find that using a box grater first speeds up the process.

Sauté the minced mushrooms in butter over medium heat. Salt them to bring out the moisture. Keep them bubbling lightly, stirring occasionally. Do this for 15-20 minutes (you can be doing other things while this is going on). The idea is to create a lovely undertone of umami. If this is too much trouble for you, and if you don't want to screw around with it, you can skip the minced/sautéed mushrooms. The dish will still be tasty.

While the mushrooms are cooking (assuming you have the ambition to use them), julienne the zucchini and summer squash with the Zyliss mandolin. WATCH YOUR FINGERS! The device is very efficient and helpful if you respect it. It includes a pusher to keep your fingers away from the blades. Please use the pusher.

Pour the canned clam sauce and canned minced clams into a separate sauce pan and warm.

When the mushrooms have lost their moisture and cooked for 15-20 minutes, raise the heat and introduce the julienned veggies to the sauté pan. Hit the veggies with salt and a drizzle of olive oil.

Using two paddles, stir/mix the veggie strands now and then for just a few minutes. You don't need to cook them very long. 2-4 minutes max.

Turn off the heat.

Put a portion of the veggies/mushroom mix into a bowl, and pour a serving of the clam sauce over them.

Eat with a soup spoon and a fork for twirling.

You're welcome.

VEGGIES SAUTÉED WITH SCHMALTZ (32)

My version of schmaltz (rendered chicken fat) comes as a by-product from roasting skin-on chicken thighs. I simply collect the liquid that is left after the roasting, and refrigerate it. It will separate into two layers when it is chilled. The top layer is delicious, chickeny fat. The bottom layer is gelatinous, flavorful goodness. You want to use this within a week.

Like most of my recipes, this one is *very* flexible. I do think that the julienned squash is important, because it adds body and texture. I use my Zyliss 2 in 1 mandolin for the julienning.

We eat this as a side dish. The gelatinous layer contributes to a wonderful broth.

INGREDIENTS:

Diced onions

Diced bell pepper

Diced or cherry or grape tomatoes

A stalk of chopped celery

Julienned zucchini or summer squash

Parsley (dried is fine)

Smoked paprika

Salt & pepper

Dash of Cajun style seasoning

Schmaltz

PROCEDURE:

Start sautéing the diced onions in plenty of the rendered chicken fat…use only the fat layer, do not include the gelatinous layer at this point.

After a few minutes add the bell pepper, tomatoes and celery.

Sauté for 5-10 minutes more.

Add the gelatinous layer.

Once the gelatin has melted, add the squash, the salt and pepper, a touch of Cajun seasoning and smoked paprika, cover and heat for 2-4 minutes. The squash doesn't take long to cook.

Serve.

WEIGHT WATCHING TIP (33)

I weigh myself every day.

At 5' 9" and 190 pounds, I am not svelte. BUT, I am stable at that weight because I keep my eye on the scale each day.

I really think that this daily monitoring is important. Sure, you'll swing a few pounds day-to-day. That's not unusual, but you know what? Seeing your weight increase more than a few pounds will give you pause. Seeing that needle edge up even a little out of your normal range will make you think about your recent intake, and you'll adjust. Maybe it was those nuts. Maybe it was that commercial yogurt. Maybe it was taking two weeks off of your exercise regimen because you pulled a muscle.

One day of weight gain isn't alarming. Two days could signal a trend. Catch this trend in the bud, Bub!

WILTED SPINACH WITH SAUTÉED ONIONS & CHEESE (34)

First there was canned spinach, then there was frozen spinach, and then…wait a minute…FIRST there was *fresh* spinach!

You are in for a pleasant surprise if you have never eaten freshly cooked spinach. It has a much deeper flavor, and is appropriately moist, not soggy.

You are in for another surprise if you have never wilted (sautéed) spinach. The initial volume looks alarmingly large, but cooks down to a handful. Believe it or not, it takes about ½ pound of fresh spinach to produce one serving of wilted spinach. So you need a large pan.

INGREDIENTS:

½ pound fresh baby spinach per person.

Finely diced yellow onion.

Grated cheese. Gruyere, or a Gruyere/Swiss blend are good.

Lemon pepper.

Salt.

Butter and olive oil.

PROCEDURE:

Finely dice the onion, add to a heated, large nonstick frying pan, add salt and sauté in a little butter and olive oil until nicely softened, about 7-10 minutes.

Remove onions to a small bowl.

Bring pan back to heat, add a bit of butter and a drizzle of olive oil, then mound the spinach into the pan. Depending on volume, you may need to cook the first batch down a bit before adding more spinach to the pan.

Turn the spinach at 15-30 second intervals (you'll soon get the timing) with a spatula, being sure to bring the bottom, wilted spinach, up to the top.

Season spinach with lemon pepper and a little salt (keep in mind that the cheese naturally has some salt).

Once the spinach is fully wilted, which won't take long, add the diced onions and grated cheese in a few layers, stirring and folding between additions.

Place in a covered dish and keep warm until served.

CONCLUSION (35)

You will have noticed by now that the premise of the Defiant Diet is pleasantly simple: Eat as little sugar and as few carbs as is practical, and eat as cleanly as possible.

Follow that premise and you automatically eliminate (or severely reduce) fast food and processed foods.

Read labels.

Eat more foods you prepare yourself.

Embrace this premise and you will be **HEALTHIER** and **HAPPIER**.

Sugar and carbs are undeniably bad for you, so avoiding them will make you healthier.

And happier? Who *wouldn't* be happier cooking and eating the recipes I've described?

Stay hungry, my friend.

THE HEALTHY COOKING APE

Proof

Made in the USA
Charleston, SC
17 January 2017

66379980R00033